Spiritual Care

A Practical Guide for Nurses

6

Spiritual Care

A Practical Guide for Nurses

Aru Narayanasamy

 Central Health Studies
Quay Publishing
BKT Information Services
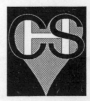

Central Health Studies is a joint venture between
Quay Publishing Ltd., Lancaster and **BKT Information Services**, Nottingham

ISBN   1 85642 054 X

British Library Cataloguing-in-Publication Data

Narayanasamy, Aru, *1951-*
  Spiritual care : a practical guide for nurses. -
  (Central health studies)
  I. Title   II. Series
  291.178321
  ISBN   1-85642-054-X

Typeset by **BKT Information Services,** Nottingham, Specialists in Desktop
Publishing, Database Development, and Electronic Media Publishing
Printed and bound in Great Britain by Biddles Ltd, Guildford and King's Lynn

Contents

Acknowledgements

My thanks are due to: Aspen Publishers inc. for permission to adapt material from *Holistic Nursing Practice*, Volume 3, p 72; Ethelrene White and Mary Wiggs for reading and commenting on the manuscript; Marj Bayne for ideas on case histories; teachers who provided the information on religious needs; Lynn Manifold, Head of the Faculty of Nursing, Mid Trent College of Nursing and Midwifery, for giving me the encouragement to write this book; my wife, Jayamani, for being a wise critic and supporter; and Gavin and Melanie for sparing their Daddy to complete this book.

Introduction

This book has been written in response to the need for a resource guide on the subject of spirituality. The purpose of this book is to provide a resource guide for nurses who want a quick guided introduction to the subject of spirituality and spiritual care.

A person functions as a whole and is made up of body, mind and spirit. In order to function as an integrated whole, the person must experience harmony between these parts. There is evidence to suggest that the spiritual part of a person receives little attention in nursing (Shelly and Fish, 1988; Carson, 1989).

Millison (1988) asserts that spirituality is an under-utilised facet of care. This book therefore aims to heighten the carers' awareness of spirituality and offers a focus on the much neglected areas of spirituality and spiritual care.

This book also offers, where relevant, further guide to reading on the subject of spirituality. Chapter One offers the reader the opportunity to understand the term "spirituality" in terms of a case illustration and activity-related work. Chapter Two provides a focus on spiritual needs and the significance of certain spiritual needs during our development and growth. Religious needs are identified in Chapter Three and guidance related to specific needs of patients from various faiths and backgrounds is provided for readers. The need for certain skills development for spiritual care is stressed and explained in Chapter Four. Chapter Five takes the reader through the process of nursing in meeting the spiritual needs of patients. This chapter includes sections on assessment, planning, implementation and evaluation of spiritual care. In Chapter Six, several case histories are provided with corresponding nursing care plans outlined. The corresponding nursing care plans apply the nursing process to the case histories. The final chapter makes reference to research related to spiritual care and acts as a valuable resource for readers looking for a starting point for research into this challenging and stimulating area of nursing.

References

CARSON, V.B. *Spiritual Dimensions of Nursing Practice*. W.B. Saunders, 1989

MILLISON, M.B., Spirituality and Caregiver, Developing an underutilised facet of care, *The American Journal of Hospice Care*, March/April 1988, pp. 3744

SHELLY, J.A and FISH, S. *Spiritual Care: The Nurse's Role*. InterVarsity Press, 1988

Chapter One:
Spirituality

Holistic approaches to health and health care require a holistic view of persons. Most of us claim our commitment to holistic care; by this we mean care of the body, mind and spirit. However, the provision of spiritual care is less than ideal in practice. This is a gross injustice to the claim that nursing fully embraces holistic care.

In a world dominated by secularism, today's focus tend to be on things that are orientated on the present, materialistic, and tangible. It is not surprising that for many, spirituality is seen as something to do with religion, whilst others may attach very little importance to it. Concern for the spiritual aspects of a person, (things that are sacred and eternal) is likely to receive less attention in our world dominated by technological advances and expectations of immediate results. Human life is governed by social, psychological, physical and spiritual influences. If we are to accept that spiritual aspects of a person are just as important as social, psychological and physical dimensions of life, then we must pay serious attention to beliefs and practices that govern individuals.

Spiritual beliefs and practices permeate the life of a person, whether in health or illness. Certain spiritual needs tend to feature during our personal development and growth. The influence of spirituality and religion is commonly seen in the following aspects of a person's life: relationships with others, living style and habits; required and prohibited behaviours; and the general frame of reference for thinking about oneself and the world. Our spirituality features during our development and growth.

In nursing a focus on the notion of totality of the person as encompassing body, mind and spirit is gaining recognition, but there is little elaboration on what is meant by spirit. This problem is further compounded by the misuse of the term spirituality, in that this word is equated to, or is applied synonymously with, institutional religion. Institutional religions usually refer (in the UK at least) to Christianity and Judaism.

What is Spirituality ?

There is no single authoritative definition of spirituality although a variety of explanation are offered in the emerging literature on this subject. As mentioned earlier, when we talk about holistic approach we mean care for the body, mind and spirit. Holistic care is a popular theme, at least, from a theoretical angle but spirituality as an aspect of nursing care is given little weight. We need to understand the concept of spirituality if we are going to offer it as a component of holistic nursing care.

Although there is an overlap between spirituality, psychology, sociology, politics and so on, it should be seen as a discipline with developing schools of theories. You will find that religious needs and spirituality are closely connected, and sometimes one finds it is difficult to make the distinction between them as one need affects the other. Please attempt Activity Number One below.

Activity One

Spend a few minutes thinking about spirituality, and then write below what you mean by the term "spirituality"?:

Feedback on activity one

When you tried to think about spirituality , perhaps, several concepts may have arisen in your mind. Your written responses may have included some or all of the following:

- A belief in God,
- A belief affecting your life and how it relates to others,
- Something not necessarily religious,
- A belief/ concept; purpose and meaning,
- Faith/ peace with oneself; a source of strength,
- Feeling of security/ to be loved,
- Philosophy of life/ death/ religion,
- Self Esteem/ Inner Self, Inner strength,
- Searching/ coping; hope,
- An idealism, a striving to be good; a trusting relationship.

History suggests that since the beginning of man/womankind spirituality has always featured in people's lives in some way or another. Spirituality is one of the fashionable words in nursing, yet like so many useful and comprehensive terms, it is not easy to define. You probably arrived at similar conclusion from the activity you had just completed.

Spirituality can be defined as:

"A quality that goes beyond religious affiliation, that strives for
inspirations, reverence, awe, meaning and purpose, even in
those who do not believe in any god. The spiritual dimension
tries to be in harmony with the universe, strives for answers

about the infinite, and comes into focus when the person faces emotional stress, physical illness or death."

(Murray and Zentner, p 259).

Spirituality equally applies to the needs of believers and non-believers and in contexts where religious beliefs may be varied. It is not uncommon for individuals with no religious allegiance to be able to relate to some spiritual or natural force, beyond the physical and self.

Spirituality is seen as an inner thing that is central to the person's being and one that makes a person unique and "tick over" as an individual. For example, I see it as my being; my inner person. It is who I am unique and alive. It is expressed through my body, my thinking, my feelings, my judgements, and my creativity. My spirituality motivates me to choose meaningful relationships and pursuits. Sometimes we desire for personal quest for meaning and purpose in life; a sense of harmonious relationship (interconnectedness) with self and others, nature, an ultimate other, and other factors which are necessary for our integrity. I would like to illustrate these points in the case of Elsie below. (The case illustration and elements of spirituality are adapted from *Holistic Nursing Practice*, 1990)

Case Illustration

Elsie looks after her elderly mother who is an invalid and has been a widow for the last ten years. She feels that it is her duty to care for her mother who is totally dependent on her. Elsie frequently says to the District Nurse that it has not always been an easy task, but she has learnt a lot in the last ten years. Through caring for her mother, she has become more appreciative of the beauty and joy in life. Elsie sees each day as new opportunity to learn and grow. The District Nurse feels that in Elsie's presence one experiences a sense of peace, since, even in the midst of difficult and trying circumstance, she affirms that life is good. Elsie says she has done some soul-searching over the last ten years and has come to know herself pretty well. She states to the District Nurse that when she felt low, she learned to "go inside myself" and always find guidance there and achieves a sense of relief and comfort. She also adds that she maintains close relationship with family and friends, with whom she shares love and support. Elsie is a keen gardener and when in her garden she feels close to the earth and to the Creator.

Several of the elements of spirituality can be illustrated in the case of Elsie:

Unfolding mystery: through life's "ups and downs" and what could be viewed as a burden, she has found meaning as peace and joy;

Inner Strength: she has developed a great sense of self awareness, which she has gained by going inside herself (a process also known as introspection) for guidance;

Harmonious interconnectedness: she has loving, supporting relationships with family and friends, a sense of knowing herself;

Source of strength and hope: the garden has become a place where she is able to express a feeling of closeness to nature and to the Creator.

It appears that spirituality is essential to our well-being and is the essence of our existence. It has to do with both solitude and corporate life including the way we think, act and feel in every day life. In essence, we can now see that it influences the whole of our lives.

Furthermore, through spirituality we give and receive love. One responds to appreciate God, other people, a sunset, a symphony, or spring. Many of us keep our spirits up in spite of adversity and it may be well because something motivates us to do so. This is because of our spirituality. Elsie's situation is a good example of spirituality as it keeps her going in spite of all the odds. We are driven forward, sometimes because of pain, sometimes in spite of pain. Spirituality permits a person to function, motivated and able to value, worship, and communicate with the holy, the transcendent.

Transcendence is as much a personal need as are physiological or psychological requirements. If we take this view, then we as nurses must regard all individuals as spiritual beings and not as a body with just physiological and psychological needs.

Spiritual Well-being

After this discussion of spirituality, let us now turn our attention to the concept of spiritual well-being. Please attempt Activity Number Two below.

Activity Two

Consider for a few minutes what you mean by spiritual well-being, and then write out your responses.

Feedback on activity

Spiritual well-being is an important facet of health and is considered as affirmation of our relationship with God/ Transcendent, self, community and environment that nurtures and keeps us as an integrated whole person. The following are features of our spiritual well-being:

- the belief in God that is fostered through communication with Supreme Being;

5

- expression of love, concern, and forgiveness for others; giving and accepting help;
- accepting and valuing of self; and
- expressing life satisfaction.

Furthermore, our spiritual well-being is usually demonstrated by our ability to find meaning and purpose in present life situations and to search for meaning and purpose in the future. It is also a state of harmonious relationship between self, others/nature, and ultimate other that is enduring throughout life and extends beyond time and space. We can attain spiritual well-being through a dynamic and integrative growth process which leads to a realization of the ultimate purpose and meaning in life.

Clearly, there is no one single authoritative definition of spirituality, although some authors have attempted to define it in broader terms. Spirituality refers to a broader dimension which is sometimes beyond the realm of subjective explanation. It is an inspirational expression as a reaction to a religious force or an abstract philosophy as defined by the individual. It is a quality that is present in believers, and even in atheists and agnostics, provided there is the opportunity to feel and express this inspirational experience according to the individuals understanding and meaning attached to this phenomenon. In the next chapter the development of spiritual needs is explored and explained.

REFERENCES

MURRAY, R.B. & ZENTNER, J.B., *Nursing Concepts for Health Promotion* Prentice Hall, 1989

FURTHER READING GUIDE

Readers wishing to explore further the concept of spirituality may find the following useful.

CARSON, V.B. *Spiritual Dimensions of Nursing Practice*, W.B. Saunders, 1989

The concept of spirituality is adequately treated in Chapter One of this book.

SHELLY, J.A. & FISH, S. *Spiritual Care: The Nurse's Role*, InterVarsity Press 1988.

Although written from a Christian perspective readers will find 'useful sections which explore the concept of spirituality. Chapters One to Three are particularly useful and assist the reader to 'grasp' the concept of spirituality. The book also includes a workbook section which contains individual exercises for developing spiritual awareness.

Chapter Two:
Spiritual Needs

As previously seen, the holistic view is that we all have needs which are regarded as social, psychological, physical and spiritual. Many of us have less trouble in identifying needs that are described as social, psychological and physical, but we struggle to identify spiritual needs.

Read the case illustration below and attempt the activity that follows.

Case Illustration

Mary, aged 78 years and widowed, lives alone and suffers from chronic arthritis. Her daughter and two sons visit her regularly and they are her constant source of support. Mary's arthritis gives her a lot of pain and sometimes she wonders why she has to suffer and tries to find meaning in her chronic disability. However, she finds meaning and hope through her prayers as she is a devoted Christian. Mary's daughter takes her to Church whenever possible, where Mary finds the companionship of her fellow churchgoers a good source of strength and support.

Her youngest son, John and his family have just returned to England after a long spell in Australia. He left England for Australia 20 years ago following an argument with his father. Mary feels guilty about the unresolved conflict between her son and husband, and feels that reconciliation should have taken place before her husband's death. She tries to seek forgiveness for both through her prayers. Mary is delighted to see her grandchildren from Australia, whom she had missed all these years, and now finds inspiration and new meaning and hope in her life as a result. Mary's renewed hope has given her inspiration to rework her goals and she finds a new purpose in her life. Her arthritis is no longer the dominant feature in her life and she is now able to resume painting, and finds satisfaction in expressing creative talent through her artistic work.

Activity: *Identify Mary's spiritual needs and list them.*

Feedback on activity: We express our spiritual needs in a variety of ways and forms. Your list of Mary's spiritual needs may include the following:

- the need for meaning and purpose
- the need for love and harmonious relationship
- the need for forgiveness
- the need for a source of hope and strength

- the need for trust
- the need for expression of personal beliefs and values
- the need for spiritual practices, expression of concept of God or Deity and creativity.

I will now expand on each of these needs:

Meaning and purpose

Many people tend to find themselves wrestling with the meaning and purpose in life during crisis, whether in health or illness. In the earlier case illustration, Mary tried to find meaning in her suffering. Meaning in this context can be defined as the reason given to a particular life experience by the individual. The search for meaning is a primary force in life. This drives us to search for meaning to life in general and discovering meaning in suffering in particular. We need to find sense out of our life and illness. Mary, in the case illustration above, found new meaning and purpose in her changed circumstances.

There is evidence to suggest that patients struggle with finding a source of meaning and purpose in their lives (Peterson and Nelson 1987; Burnard,1990). It is suggested that people with a sense of meaning and purpose survive more readily in very difficult circumstances and these include illness and suffering. There is some truth in the expression that he who has a "why" to life can bear with almost any "how". We approach the task of life in a variety of ways and our ability to cope with crisis varies. We can find meaning and purpose in the experience of suffering. There is a distinction between the religious and the apparently non-religious person in the way they approach spirituality, that is the religious person experiences his existence not merely as a task but as a mission, and is aware of his taskmaster, the source of his mission. That source is a Supreme Being which for Christians is God, for Muslims, Allah, and for Hindus and Bhuddists, the Transcendent.

In crisis, such as bereavement, people frequently experience meaninglessness, and express a sense of bewilderment and loss of meaning in life. For example, the person with a diagnosis of HIV infection, the survivor of a traumatic road accident, a parent grieving over the death of a child, the patient in a mental health unit, may all cry out for help in search of meaning, and desperately seek someone who will give them attention and time in their exploration of meaning and purpose. The nurse is very often the nearest person to whom sufferers can reach out.

In a person searching for meaning and purpose, there may be a need for exploration of spiritual issues. In some instances the person in search of spirituality may want to talk about religious feelings or lack of them. The person may not be asking for advice or opinions, but just for an opportunity to talk about feelings, to express doubts and anguish. Such opportunity for expression can bring about clarity and a renewed sense of meaning and purpose.

Those who have strong religious conviction and sense God, still need encouragement to adapt to unexpected changes. They are likely to experience hope even when their usual support systems let them down since their experience of God reassures them that God will never fail them. However the nurse may have to act as a catalyst in helping patients to find meaning and purpose in crisis by establishing their relationship with God.

ove and Harmonious Relationship

Our need for love and harmonious relationship goes hand in hand with a need for meaning and purpose. The need for love is one of the fundamental human needs (Maslow, 1968) which last throughout life (from childhood to old age). A spiritually distressed person requires unconditional love, that is love that has no strings attached to it. This is sometimes referred as "in spite of" love. The spiritually distressed person does not have to earn it by being good or attractive or wealthy. The person is simply loved for the way he or she is, regardless of faults or ignorance or bad habits or deeds. The spiritual needs of Mary, the lady in the illustration above, were met by her relationships with her family and fellow churchgoers.

The manifestations of the need for love are self pity, depression, insecurity, isolation, and fear. These are indicators of a need for love from oneself, other people and God. The person receiving this kind of love experiences feelings of self-worth, joy, security, belonging, hope and courage.

The following can be identified as signs of spiritual problems in a person who needs to receive love:

- worries about how the rest of the family will manage after his or her death;
- expression of feelings of a loss of faith in God;
- reluctance to discuss feelings about dying with persons who are close to one;
- not calling on others when help is needed;
- expression of fear of tests and diagnosis;
- expression of feeling lack of support from others;
- conforming behaviour, reflecting that of a 'good' patient or person
- refusal to cooperate with health care regime;
- expression of guilt feelings;

- thoughts of confession and feelings about shameful events;
- expression of anger with self/others;
- expressions of ambivalent feelings toward God;
- expression of despondency during illness/ hospitalisation;
- expression of resentment toward God;
- expression of loss of self-value due to decreasing physical capacity;
- expression of fear of God's anger.

The spiritually distressed person also has a need to give love, which may be indicated, for example, by worries about the financial status of family during hospitalisation/ separation from family and worries about separation from others by death.

Forgiveness

We saw in Mary's case the need for forgiveness and this is one of the principal causes of spiritual distress. A person who experiences spiritual distress expresses feelings of guilt and therefore requires the opportunity for forgiveness. Mary sought forgiveness for her son and husband through her prayers. Guilt often emerges when people experience the feeling that they have failed to live up to their own expectation or the expectations of others. For example, we may first experience guilt as a child when our behaviour does not measure up to the standards set for us by our parents. We contradict them and do the very things we are told not to do. Guilt breeds in us in the form of regrets, not only for the things we have done but for our failures in many things. Unresolved conflicts in relationships can result in feelings of guilt.

The feelings of guilt may be expressed as feelings of paranoia, hostility, worthlessness, defensiveness, withdrawal, psychosomatic complaints, rationalisations, criticism of self, others and God, and scapegoating. Forgiveness may bring a feeling of joy, peace and elation, and a sense of renewed self-worth. It seems that confession of sin is one way in which some people achieve a sense of their God's forgiveness.

Hope and Strength

Hope is seen by psychologists and sociologists as necessary for life and without it we begin to die (Simsen, 1988). For many of us our sense of hope can be a powerful motivator in enabling an open attitude toward new ways of coping. Mary, in the case illustration, achieves new hope and strength from reconciliation with her son and his family. The spiritually distressed person may experience a feeling of hopelessness. The hopeless person may see no way out; there may be no other possibilities other than those dreaded.

We met in Mary's situation her new goals and a renewed purpose as result of her son's arrival from Australia. We thrive on good relationship with others and this is another facet of our hope. This includes relationships with others, oneself, and the world, where a person believes and what is desired is possible.

According to Soeken and Carson (1987): "Ultimate hope resides in God and belief that the Supreme Being will impart meaning to individual lives and sufferings. Both components of hope are important for the patient with chronic illness" (pp. 610). Hope is also necessary for future plans. Further needs of our hope include seeking support, love and the stability provided by important relationships in our life, and putting into action future plans. In the case illustration, Mary successfully achieves all of these through her loved ones and friends. If the patient believes in God, then hope in God is important. This hoping in God is the ultimate source of strength and supersedes all aspirations that are transitional.

Hope is closely related to our need for a source of strength. A source of hope provides the strength that we may need. A source of strength gives us the courage needed to face innumerable odds in crisis. The main source of hope and strength is found by individuals who pray because of their faith in God or the Transcendent. Haase's (1987) study found that the subjects concurred that belief in the power of prayer helped them cope with medical procedures and opportunities to express their faith helped them to resolve the situation they described. For some communication with God and prayer is a source of strength. For most of us, a message of hope provides new energy, strength, and courage to preserve or revise goals or plan and these were apparent in Mary's situation.

Trust

We feel secure when we can establish a trusting relationship with others. The spiritually distressed person needs an environment that conveys a trusting relationship. Such an environment is one which demonstrates that carers make themselves accessible to others, both physically and emotionally. Trusting is the ability to place confidence in the trustworthiness of others and this is essential for spiritual health and to total well-being. Learning to trust in an environment which is alien could be a daunting task and not an easy skill to accomplish.

Personal beliefs and values

The opportunity to express personal values and beliefs is a known spiritual need. In this sense, spirituality refers to anything that a person considers to be of highest value in life. Mary shares her beliefs with her companions at the church and expresses these through her prayers. Her spiritual needs in these areas are met easily through the support of her family. Personal values which are highly regarded by an individual may include, for example, beliefs of a formalised religion, whereas for others they may be a set of very personal philosophical statements, or perhaps a physical activity, e.g. working for voluntary or charity organizations.

Spiritual Practices, Concept of God/Deity, and Creativity

The concept of God or Deity may be an important function in the personal life of a person. The need to carry out spiritual practices concerning God or Deity may be too daunting for the person if the opportunity is not available or the environment is alien or unreceptive to this need.

Our creative needs may feature in spirituality. Mary fulfils the spiritual need of creativity through her paintings. A religious minister uses the arts as an avenue to the Spirit; actors, writers, musicians, and artists of a university are invited to exhibit their work and give performances at his Connecticut hospice (Wald, 1989).

HUMAN DEVELOPMENT AND SPIRITUAL NEEDS

Certain spiritual needs tend to feature at different times during our personal development and growth. During infancy, trust is a major spiritual need; during childhood we learn to understand concepts about religion from our parents and people close to us, and in adolescence there is a tendency to search for meaning and value in life.

Fears can be regarded as clues to children's spiritual needs, and such fears may include sudden movements, loud noises, loss of support, pain, fear of strangers or strange objects, heights, or anticipated unpleasant situations. Unmet needs for love and relationship may manifest as those fears. So, meeting the infant's need for basic trust has an impact on spiritual development.

During childhood one learns to understand religious concepts from parents and other people in his environment. The child's inquisitive mind may prompt him to ask questions about basic issues of life, for example: "What is God?", "Why doesn't John have a Christmas Tree?" and "Why did Granny go to heaven?"

The spiritual needs of the child include need for love and security. Also, the child is likely to imitate his parent's faith, and some of his concept of faith may be based on fantasy.

The child also learns to recognise what is "Good" or "Bad" from his parents and other significant people around him. During crises, such as admission to hospital, the child often has a great difficulty with verbal expression of his spiritual concerns. The death of a loved one may make this even more of a problem. The child does not understand that death is universal, inevitable and irreversible.

In adolescence the search for meaning and value in life may feature as a spiritual need. Problems may arise as a result of conflicts within the family because of moral standards set by parents. Conflicts may arise as a result of double standards: behaviour expected by parents may conflict with the behaviour of parents. Because of these conflicts, the adolescent's source of strength and support could come from his/her peer group.

During young adulthood one seeks for trust, for love, for hope, and forgiveness. There may be an experience of tension, expectations and spiritual struggle. It is also a time for restructuring of religious, moral and ethical values. During the stage of young adulthood there may be a period in which reorientation and growth in the spiritual realm takes place.

In middle years, the questioning of life precipitated by the death of parents or peers, children leaving home, plans for retirement, or an awareness of one's physical failings may feature. The four common spiritual needs in middle-age are:

1) The need for meaning and purpose in life;

2) The need to be forgiven;

3) The need to receive love; and

4) The need for hope and creativity.

In old age, a stock of life's successes and failures is often taken together with a renewal of religious faith and spiritual beliefs. Many people experience a more positive self concept as a result of accomplishment and worth. Some may find great social and spiritual fulfilment in having some kind of religious affiliation. Religious ceremonies such as marriages, baptism, and burials may become significant. Religious expression may be fulfilled by attendances at the church or place of worship. Church or religious affiliation promotes feelings of hope and purpose to life for many older people.

SUMMARY

In this chapter an attempt has been made to identify spiritual needs which include the need for meaning and purpose; the need for love and harmonious relationships; the need for forgiveness; the need for a source of hope and strength; the need for trust; the need for expression of personal beliefs and values; and the need for spiritual practice, expression of concept of God or Deity and creativity. These are by no means exclusive, but commonly recognised as within the province of nursing to be incorporated into care plans as part of spiritual care of patients. Finally, certain spiritual needs as a feature of our development were outlined.

REFERENCES

BURNARD, P. Learning to care for the spirit, *Nursing Standard*, 24 Jan 1990, 4(18), pp. 3839

HAASE J.E. Components of Courage in Chronically Ill Adolescents: A phenomenological Study *Advanced Nursing Science*, 1987 (9) pp. 64

MASLOW, A.R. *Toward a Psychology of Being* D. Van Nostrand, 1968

PETERSON, E. & NELSON, K. How to Meet Your Clients' Spiritual Needs *Journal of Psychosocial Nursing*, May 1987, 25(5), pp. 348

SIMSEN, B. Nursing the Spirit, *Nursing Times*, 1988, 84(37) , pp. 31–35

SOEKEN, K.L. & CARSON, Y.J. Responding to the spiritual needs of the Chronically Ill? *Nursing Clinics of North America*, Sept. 1987, 22(3), pp. 603–611

WALD, F.S. The Widening Scope of Spiritual Care, *American Journal of Hospice Care*, July/August 1989, pp. 40-43

Chapter Three:
Resource Guide to Religious Faiths and Needs

As we have seen earlier, spirituality and religion are inextricably connected and sometimes it is difficult to separate the two. In order to provide a satisfactory spiritual care, we have to understand the religious needs of patients who have strong religious faiths. Religion is defined as:

> "A belief in a supernatural or divine force that has power over
> the universe and commands worship and obedience; a system
> of beliefs; a comprehensive code of ethics or philosophy; a set
> of practices that are followed; a church affiliation; the con-
> scious pursuit of any object the person holds as supreme."

(Murray and Zentner, pp. 259).

In many hospitals, particularly in inner cities, nursing involves caring for patients from a variety of religious and cultural background. An understanding of these differing religious needs is an important prerequisite for spiritual care.

Activity: *Consider for a few minutes the different faiths of your patients or of people you know, and then write down below the faiths you have identified.*

Feedback on activity: Compare your list with the table that is given overleaf. Your list may have matched with religions indicated in this table. The table demonstrates that the UK is a pluralistic society when it comes to religions.

It is beyond the scope of this book to provide the wider coverage that all religions rightly deserve. However, if you require some insights into the religions of the United Kingdom, a brief outline of each religion is given, together with a reading guide.

Spiritual Care

Table

APPROXIMATE COMMUNITY SIZES (throughout the whole of the UK)

	1975	1980		1975	1980
	millions	millions		millions	millions
Church of England	27.5	26.6[1]	Jews	0.4	0.4
Other Episcopal	0.7[1]	0.7[1]	Church of Scientology	0.3	0.5
Baptists	0.6[2]	0.6[1]	Other churches		
Methodists	1.5	1.5	(JWs, Mormons etc.)	0.7[1]	0.7[1]
Presbyterian[4]	1.9[1]	1.70[1]	Hindus	0.2[1]	0.3[1]
Roman Catholics	5.2[2]	5.2	Muslims	0.5[2]	1.0
Other Trinitarian Churches	1.10[1]	1.3[1]	Sikhs 0.2	0.4	
			Other religions	0.1[1]	0.2[1]
Total Christian Churches	38.5[2]	37.6	Total Other	24.2[2]	3.5
			Total All Religions	40.9[2]	41.1
			Percentage of Population[3]	73%	74%

[1]Estimate
[2]Revised figure
[3]UK Population 56.0m in 1975, 55.9m in 1980
[4]Congregational figures now included with 'other trinitarian churches'

Source: Brierley (Ed.), *UK Christian Handbook 1983*, London: Evangelical Alliance, Bible Society, MARC Europe, 1982.

READING GUIDE

CHRISTIANITY

Notes

Christianity in some form will probably be the religion with which most nurses and students of nursing who read this book are familiar. Christianity is the religion that is based on Jesus Christ. It is the largest and most universal religion of more than one billion believers. Beliefs of Christianity are explained within the Old and New Testament books of the Holy Scriptures. These include belief in God, Jesus Christ, the Holy Spirit, Sin, Redemption, Salvation, and Retribution or a final accounting with God at the end of life.

16

Reading List

Readers wishing a greater insight into Christianity and its various denominations may find the following book useful:

FELLOW, W. *Religions: East and West* New York: Holt, Rinehart and Winston, 1978

This book also includes details of other religions (see below).

If you require further information on Christian spirituality, you may consult the Dictionary edited by Gordon Wakefield, *A Dictionary of Christian Spirituality*, SCM Press, 1983.

Surprisingly, this book also has good sections on Islam, Hinduism, Buddhism, and Rastafarianism. The last is particularly useful, as information on Rastafarianism is particularly hard to find.

A book edited by Terence Thomas offers some perspectives on the religious beliefs and practices of the British.

THOMAS, T.(Ed.) *The British, Their Religious Beliefs and Practices (1880-1986)*. London: Routledge, 1988

This book also has valuable sections on statistics related to church attendances and to other religions.

If you are looking for nursing texts which make specific reference to Christianity, the following may be consulted:

MURRAY, R.B. & ZENTNER, J.P. *Nursing Concepts for Health Promotion* Prentice Hall, 1989

This book is written in the North American context, which should be born in mind when reading it.

McGILLOWAY, D. & MYCO, F. *Nursing and Spiritual Care* Harper & Row, 1985.

Chapter Six looks at the Christian Patient and the role of the chaplain.

CARSON, V.B. *Spiritual Dimensions of Nursing Practice* W.B. Saunders Co., 1989

Chapter Four provides insight into Western Spirituality and Health Care.

RUMBOLD, G. *Ethics in Nursing Practice* Bailliere Tindall, 1986

Chapter 2 provides a brief outline of some of the main religions with particular reference to ethical issues in health care.

ISLAM

Notes

Islam was originated in the Middle East at the beginning of the Seventh Century by the Prophet Muhammad. It is the youngest of the major world religions. Muslims believe in one God, "Allah" and Muhammad, His Prophet provides the key to Moslem beliefs. Muslim means "peaceful submission to God's will". The teachings of Prophet Muhammad were recorded in the Qur'an (or Koran). Islam is one of the major religions of the world and there is a great deal of similarity in the practices and beliefs of all muslims, however, some differences exist in the interpretations and explanation of the Koran by the main (two) sects in Islam—the Sunni Muslims and the Shia Muslims (McAvoy & Donaldson, 1990)

Reading List

The following are useful reading resources on Islam:

FELLOW, W. *Religions: East and West* New York: Holt, Rinehart and Winston, 1978

This book gives a good historical background to this religion and includes the main tenets of its faith.

HOLROYDE, P., MOHAMMED I. AND VOHRA D.K. *East comes West* London: Community Relations Commission, 1974.

The section on Islam will give you a good insight. It is clear and thorough enough, if you are seeking an understanding of this religion.

McAVOY B.R. & DONALDSON, L.J. (Eds.) *Health Care for Asia* Oxford Medical Publications, 1990.

This book will provide a thorough understanding of cultural and religious aspects of Asians in Britain. There are good sections on Islam and the needs of the Muslim patient throughout the book. It is one of the best books available on health care of Asians.

For guidance on the nursing care of Muslims, the following may also be useful:

MURRAY, R.B. & ZENTNER, J.P. *Nursing Concepts for Health Promotion* Prentice Hall, 1989

McGILLOWAY, D. & MYCO, F. *Nursing and Spiritual Care* Harper & Row, 1985.

Chapter Nine provides perspectives of Muslim patients.

CARSON, V.B. *Spiritual Dimensions of Nursing Practice* W.B. Saunders Co., 1989

UDAISM

otes

Modern Judaism has three main divisions: Orthodox, Conservative and Reform. Reform Judaism is somewhat more liberal than the other two divisions in its beliefs and practices. Orthodox Judaism is the stricter of the other two, and adherents believe that God gave the law and that it should be followed precisely as written. Certain beliefs are shared by almost all Jews:

- God is the one and only God,
- He is holy, sacred, and separate from the world and people,
- By his word he creates, rules, and judges the world and people, and speaks to Israel and all people,
- He will bring history to fulfilment in the messianic age.

The theory and practice of Jewish ethics include:

- that the moral law comes from God, as such it is absolute, universal, revealed, and humane,
- the law consists in the Commandments of God, which are interpreted by the Rabbi, to be studied and followed by all, as a blessing for them and for the world.

eading List

FELLOW, W. *Religions: East and West* New York: Holt, Rinehart and Winston, 1978

If you need further information on Jewish Spirituality, you may also consult the Dictionary edited by Gordon Wakefield, *A Dictionary of Christian Spirituality*, SCM Press, 1983.

If you are looking for nursing texts which make specific reference to Judaism, then the following may be useful to you:

MURRAY, R.B. & ZENTNER, J.P. *Nursing Concepts for Health Promotion* Prentice Hall, 1989

McGILLOWAY, D. & MYCO, F. *Nursing and Spiritual Care* Harper & Row, 1985.

Chapter Seven provides insights into caring for Jewish patients.

CARSON, V.B. *Spiritual Dimensions of Nursing Practice* W.B. Saunders Co., 1989

Chapter Four provides insights into Judaism.

HINDUISM

Notes

The Hindus believe in one God, who can be worshipped in many different forms, the important ones being Brahma (the Creator), Vishnu (the Preserver), and Shiva (the Destroyer). Many Hindus carry out prayers in Shrines at their homes in front of various pictures of incarnations of the Deities, where incense is burnt. Beliefs in non-violence and reincarnation are held.

Reincarnation is the cycle of birth and re-birth and based on the notion that all persons are responsible for their actions in each life, and undergo a cycle of rebirth until their lifestyles raise above their previous lives and unite them with God. Status and conditions in each life are determined by behaviour in the last life.

Religion is a way of life for the Hindus and one that is constant and pervades all aspects of their lives. Bhagavad-Gita is a sacred Hindu text and the Ramayana and Mahabhrata are the two great epics in Hinduism.

Reading List

If you are looking for some insights into Hinduism, the book by Geoffrey Parrinder is useful:

PARRINDER, G. *Asian Religions* London: Sheldon Press, 1968.

FELLOW, W. *Religions: East and West* New York: Holt, Rinehart and Winston, 1978

This book gives a good historical background to this religion and includes the main tenets of Hinduism.

HOLROYDE, P., MOHAMMED I. AND VOHRA D.K. *East comes West* London: Community Relations Commission, 1974.

Easy to read material on Hinduism is provided.

McAVOY B.R. & DONALDSON, L.J. (Eds.) *Health Care for Asia* Oxford Medical Publications, 1990.

This book is very informative on health care of Asians who are Hindus.

All the titles mentioned so far provide good starting points before you look at some of the more advanced materials on the subject.

A word of caution: some of the concepts can be difficult to grasp initially, but if you are interested it is worthwhile pursuing your reading.

You will also find good sections on the nursing care of Hindu patients in the following books:

MURRAY, R.B. & ZENTNER, J.P. *Nursing Concepts for Health Promotion* Prentice Hall, 1989

Chapter 9.

McGILLOWAY, D. & MYCO, F. *Nursing and Spiritual Care* Harper & Row, 1985.

Chapter Eight provides perspectives on Hindu patients.

CARSON, V.B. *Spiritual Dimensions of Nursing Practice* W.B. Saunders Co., 1989

Chapter 5

IKHISM

otes

Sikhism, a religion founded by Guru Nanak (1469–1538), is based on the teachings of ten Gurus. The Sikh Holy book is the Guru Granth Sahab, which is a collection of the writings of the ten Gurus. Sikhism is based on one God, with great importance given to worship to, and to a personal relationship with, God. The Sikhs believe in reincarnation but reject the notion of caste on the grounds that all people are equal. The Gurdwara (temple) provides a common centre for group worship and acts as a meeting place for the community. There are five signs which are significant to Sikhism.

- **Kara** – a metal bangle which is usually not removed, worn by men and women,
- **Kesh** – uncut hair,
- **Kangha** – the comb used to secure long hair under a turban,
- **Kirpan** – a small symbolic dagger; and
- **Kaccha** – a sacred undergarment.

Spiritual Care

'Taking Amrit' is special devotion in Sikhism in that Sikhs undertake this are known as 'Amrit Dari' and promise to wear the five signs of Sikhism, carry out special prayers, not eat meat, and attend the gurdwara every day. The Sikhs use the title Singh (for males), and Kaur (for females).

Reading List

HOLROYDE, P., MOHAMMED I. AND VOHRA D.K. *East comes West* London: Community Relations Commission, 1974.

Easy to read material on Sikhism is given.

McAVOY B.R. & DONALDSON, L.J. (Eds.) *Health Care for Asia* Oxford Medical Publications, 1990.

This book is very informative on health care of Asians who are Sikhs.

PARRINDER, G. *Asian Religions* London: Sheldon Press, 1968.

BUDDHISM

Notes

Buddhism was founded by Gautama in India who lived from 643 to 563 B.C. Buddhism embraces the following: Four Noble Truths and the Noble Eightfold Path.

The Four Noble Truths are:

1. Suffering is universal;
2. The cause of suffering is craving, or selfish desire;
3. The use of suffering is the elimination of craving; and
4. The way to eliminate craving is to follow the middle way, a technique which embodies the Noble Eightfold Path.

The Path consists of:

1. Right knowledge
2. Right intention
3. Right Speech
4. Right conduct
5. Right means of livelihood

6.   Right effort

7.   Right mindfulness

8.   Right concentration.

The Buddhist strives to achieve an impersonal ultimate reality through a purifying life of ethical thinking and by carrying out good deeds. The ultimate goal of a Buddhist is the achievement of Nirvana—a state of liberation, i.e. freeing one from suffering, death and rebirth, and all other worldly bonds.

It is the highest, transcendent consciousness.

Buddhists are said to believe in reincarnation, but they do not accept the Hindus' view of the transmigration of souls through various forms of life. Monastic life is important in Buddhism, in which withdrawal from and relinquishing the eating of meat and owning of personal property is possible. Many Buddhist youngsters and men spend a part of their lives as monks, but most return to mainstream life. Essentially, most Buddhists are compassionate, avoid killing animals, and may be vegetarians.

Some say it is the gentlest of religions. Buddhism has spread to all continents and its dominating influence is found in Japan, Manchuria, Mongolia, China, Tibet, Burma, Thailand, Kampuchea and Sri Lanka. It has encouraged humanity in the form of tolerance, non-violence, respect for the individual, love of nature, and the spiritual equality of human beings. There is a variation in the way the religion is understood and practised among Buddhists.

eading Guide

The following books refer to Buddhism:

MURRAY, R.B. & ZENTNER, J.P. *Nursing Concepts for Health Promotion* Prentice Hall, 1989.

Chapter 9.

PARRINDER, G. *Asian Religions* London: Sheldon Press, 1968.

FELLOW, W. *Religions: East and West* New York: Holt, Rinehart and Winston, 1978.

This book outlines the origins and development of Buddhism.

urther resources

Information on special considerations when nursing patients of various faiths is outlined in the appendix.

Final Note

In a guide such as this it is impossible to provide the wider and deeper coverage that all religions deserve, and if there is any inaccuracy in the guidance notes related to readings/resources on religions, I apologise sincerely in advance. The guide is, as you may have realised, an attempt to optimise the holistic approach to caring for patients from a variety of backgrounds.

References

MURRAY, R.B. & ZENTNER, J.P. *Nursing Concepts for Health Promotion* Prentice Hall, 1989.

McAVOY B.R. & DONALDSON, L.J. (Eds.) *Health Care for Asia* Oxford Medical Publications, 1990.

Appendix

Specific Religious Needs of Patients

Roman Catholic

Birth   If it is suspected that life cannot be maintained, if possible summon the R.C. Chaplain. Where time does not allow for this, the Catholic or non-Catholic nurse may carry out the Baptism. This is done by pouring a small amount of water over the head three times saying these words: "[*Name of Baby*], I baptise you in the name of the Father and of the Son and of the Holy Spirit". It is usual to give the mother a small baptismal certificate. It should be noted in the Hospital Register and with the local Catholic Priest.

If a child is stillborn, a baptism must also be carried out as above by the senior nurse or catholic nurse, if available, who was present at the birth. This reassures the grieving mother and father.

Abortion/   Catholic teaching has always been to uphold human life.
Family   Every human life has a divine right to live and this also goes
Planning   for the foetus in the mother's womb. That foetus has a right to be born and to live. For this reason, the abortion is forbidden

by the Roman Catholic Church, whatever the circumstances. On the odd occasion where there may be problems as to whether to save the life of the mother-to-be or the life of the child in her womb, the Catholic stand is firmly on the side of the unborn child, but every aid must also be used to save the life of the mother.

The question of family planning is regarded by the Catholic church as being something unnatural. The church realises that often there can be all sorts of difficulties facing the couple who wish for various reasons to resort to any sort of family planning. But again, the church being invested with the authority from Christ himself, forbids family planning in the main as it regards the question of LIFE as something God-given which only he can give or take away. No man has such authority.

Transfusion   No objections.

Diet   May vary according to individual's interpretation of needs. May wish to abstain from certain foods, e.g Good Friday or other holy days.

Death   'Sacrament of anointing the sick' This should be administered at the earliest opportunity to a seriously ill patient who may eventually recover to full health and also to those seriously ill who are going to die. Often a Hospital Chaplain will be able to judge from his regular visits if, in his opinion, the patient may or will benefit form receiving the Sacrament. The earlier the Chaplain is informed the better for the patient and his/her family. A patient who has just died may still be given the Sacrament, so again it is imperative to notify the Chaplain. A record of the administered Sacrament should be noted by the ward staff.

nglican

Birth   Parents are responsible for requesting emergency Baptism, but in their absence a nurse may be the minister of Baptism and subsequently the Chaplain should be informed. The question of ultimate salvation or the provision of a Christian funeral does not depend on whether or not Baptism has taken place.

The form of Baptism to be taken is similar to as already previously documented.

Abortion/ Family Planning

The Church of England upholds the sanctity of human life and in the case of abortion everything possible should be done to preserve the lives of mother and child. In both cases the final decision is left to the person's individual conscience.

Transfusion No objection.

Diet

No particular rules. Some people may wish to abstain from certain foods at certain times, e.g. Good Friday or other holy days.

Death

Some practising Anglicans may appreciate the presence of their Parish Priest to administer sacraments of Communion, anointing or laying on of hands or bedside prayers. If a Chaplain is not available and prayers are requested then it may be helpful, if a nurse so wishes, to say the Lord's Prayer and make the sign of the cross on the patient's forehead.

Notes

Many people are nominal Church of England members and much documentation is foreign to them. Even so they may desire the appropriate prayer at the nurses/patients/relatives request. Hospital Chaplains are a good source for expert advice in the care of Christian patients and all are within the reach of carers.

Buddhist

Birth

Generally no specific rules but may not allow baby to be washed.

Abortion/ Family Planning

Very liberal attitude to contraception and abortion. No history of opposition.

Transfusion Generally accepted.

Diet Mainly vegetarian. Some 'fasting' days.

Death   Allow quietness and privacy for meditation. State of mind at death should be calm. The Buddhist believes that one must be prepared mentally for a state that would be conducive for a good rebirth. There is the belief that in facing death one must remain watchful and alert, to resist distraction and confusion, to be lucid and calm. Do not wash body. Do not move body before priest arrives if possible. Cremation is common.

Other   It should be noted that there are various sects and nationalities. Individual needs to be assessed accordingly.

Hindu

Birth   Mother may be required to rest for 40 days.

Abortion/ Family Planning   Hindu women feel that they have a duty to produce a son. Needs of the family more important than those of society. May be against abortion.

Transfusion   Generally accepted

Diet   The cow is a sacred animal and is never eaten. Many are vegetarian. Strict dietary regulations vary with each person.

Death   Hindu priest may be needed to perform certain rituals and blessings. Nursing staff can wash the body. Cremation as usual. The eldest son is responsible for funeral arrangements.

Other   The Hindu faith is centred on the transmigration of the soul with indefinite reincarnation. As a soul moves from body to body it hopes to become purer and purer until it reaches God.

Jew

Birth   Many visitors. Circumcision on eighth day.

Abortion/ Family Planning   Family planning permitted in some cases. Abortion may be considered.

Transfusion   Generally accepted. (But some restrictions on transplants.)

27

Diet   Kosher prepared meals. Strict about food preparation if orthodox.

Death   Body not to be touched by hospital staff. Body washed and
shrouded only by Rabbi. Funeral within 24 hours. Saturday—
Sabbath—day of rest.

Other   Degree of orthodoxy varies; individual needs to be assessed
accordingly.

Muslim ✓

Birth   May refuse internal examination. Circumcision prayer recited
to baby as soon as possible.

Abortion/   Not generally disapproved of, but Muslim women think it is
Family   their duty or role in life to bear children.
Planning

Transfusion   Generally accepted.

Diet   Muslims eat only 'halal' meal. May be vegetarian. Food regulations are strict; no pork, no alcohol. Observe Ramadan.

Death   Opposed to post mortems. Must adhere to specific patient's
religious duties. Koran recited by a relative. Family attend to
duties while conforming to legal regulations. Usual for family
to wash and prepare body; if not, other people wear gloves.
Burial within 24 hours.

Other   Belief that everyone is accountable to God for what he does on
earth and when he dies he will be judged or punished in life
hereafter. Patient will want to face 'Mecca'. A local Imam
(Spiritual leader) may be contacted for advice.

Care of Women – women are modest and frequently wear
clothes that cover all of the body. Modesty should be respected
as much as possible during medical examination.

Sikh

Birth	Similar to Hindu.
Abortion/ Family Planning	Often same problems about contraception and abortion apply as Hindus.
Transfusion	Generally accepted.
Diet	Fork forbidden. May be vegetarian.
Death	There are five traditional symbolic marks which all practising Sikhs should wear (as indicated earlier). It could cause distress for any of these to be removed from the dying. No objection to hospital staff handling the body.
Other	Their faith is a combination of elements of both Hindu and Moslem beliefs but tends to be more flexible.

Christian Scientist

Birth	Generally employ the use of a qualified doctor or midwife for the delivery of a child.
Abortion/ Family Planning	Christian Scientists are generally anti-abortion and anti-family planning.
Transfusion	Blood transfusions for Christian scientist avoided where possible for adults. May be accepted for children.
Diet	Avoid tobacco and alcohol. No intake of drugs.
Death	No special rites, but Christian Science burial service required.

Church of Jesus Christ of Latter Day Saints (Mormon)

Birth	Blessed at birth. Baptised at 8 years of age.

Abortion/ Family Planning   Abortion/family planning not generally accepted or recommended. Advise must be sought from Church accordingly and may be accepted for health reasons.

Transfusion   Accepted.

Diet   No drinks containing caffeine/alcohol. Drugs taken only on medical advise.

Death   Church to be contacted. Burial recommended. Elders available for 'blessing for health' and sick patients.

Jehovah's Witness

Birth   No special treatment. In emergencies it may not be advisable to give blood but can be given at discretion of Medical Officer responsible in case of emergencies.

Abortion/ Family Planning   Family planning—no objections; up to individual conscience of witness. Coil unsuitable. Abortion—all life is viewed as precious. The biblical view of abortion is that of murder, except in case of 'inevitable abortion'.

Transfusion   Adults—no transfusion—will accept plasma expanders. In emergencies, it may be advisable not to give blood, but can be given at the discretion of Medical Officer responsible. No longer need a court order to empower transfusion

Diet   Meat prepared in a special way. Advised not to eat black pudding.

Death   No other organs to be removed either for implants or experimentation. No special procedure expected.

Other   Jehovah's Witnesses carry a 'Medical Alert' card which is a signed, legal document. No participation would be expected in religious festivals and communion. For further information contact patient's own church.

Chapter Four:
Skills Development for Spiritual Care

As well as a sufficient knowledge about spiritual needs and problems, a nurse needs to develop skills of self awareness, communication (such as listening), trust building, giving hope, and acting as a catalyst for patients, to assist him/her in meeting patients' spiritual needs.

SELF AWARENESS

Before we can instigate effective spiritual care, we must know and understand our own level of spiritual awareness. An examination of our personal beliefs and values is a necessary part of spiritual care. The nurse who has a positive attitude to spiritual health is likely to be sensitive to any problem a patient has concerning spirituality. A continuous examination of our own personal spiritual beliefs, enables us (nurses included) to appreciate that everybody does not share the same faith. An awareness of our own prejudices and biases will ensure that we do not impose our own values and beliefs, especially spiritual doctrines, on others. Self awareness should enable the nurse to adopt a non-judgemental approach and avoid taking any steps that could lead to accusations of trying to proselytize. It is likely that a person who has developed self awareness will show more tolerance, acceptance and respect for other people's spirituality.

The benefits of self awareness are stressed here, but it is a skill that has to be acquired and continuously developed. In this section self awareness will be explained and a method for developing it will be outlined. Self awareness is an acknowledgement of our own feeling and behaviours, accepting and under-standing or accepting to understand these in ourselves. Self awareness can be elaborated as an acknowledgement of our:

- values, attitudes, prejudices, beliefs, assumptions, and feelings;
- personal motives and needs and the extent to which these are being met;
- degree of attention to others;
- genuineness and investment of self, and how the above might have an effect on others;
- intentional and unconscious use of self.

It is widely acknowledged that training in self awareness is a fundamental process before one understands others. According to Burnard (1985), to become aware of, and to have deeper understanding of ourselves is to have a sharper and clearer picture of what is happening to others. Limited awareness of ourselves may mean remaining blind to others. The first step to being self aware is to examine oneself, as stressed earlier.

We can develop self awareness by various means. However, the methods used for increasing our awareness must contain the facets of inner search and observations of others.

One simple method of enhancing our self awareness is the process of noticing what we are doing, the process of self monitoring; all that is involved here is staying conscious of what you are doing and what is happening to you. To put it another way, you 'stay awake' and develop the skill of keeping your attention focused on your actions, both verbal and non-verbal.

Assessment of our present understanding of knowledge, skills and the learning of new materials, skills and techniques will be heavily influenced by our degree of self awareness. We are most likely to lose control of our self development if we remain blind to the need to increase our self awareness.

Without self awareness, we cannot be in control of our own development:

- we cannot identify key performance areas;
- we cannot analyse our own performance, or identify concrete objectives;
- we cannot make action plans to help our own development; and
- we cannot monitor our own progress.

An increase in our self awareness is not only the beginning of wisdom then, but also the growth of our own personal and professional effectiveness. We can help to increase our self awareness by evaluating ourselves, by asking questions such as:

- how much time do I invest in reflecting about myself?
- how reassured am I that I have a reasonable understanding of myself?
- how do I see myself, and how do I feel about myself?
- what are my significant strengths and weaknesses?
- do I really face up to the truth about myself, or do I try to hide the truth about me from myself?

Other methods of developing our self awareness are through introspection, through experience, and through feedback:

1.   Introspection:

Meditation and yoga can be a useful way of developing self awareness using the introspection method. Simple breathing and meditation techniques are sufficient for this purpose. Meditation and yoga serve another useful purpose in that these techniques can be useful methods of dealing with job-related stress. Becoming aware of and consciously noting experiences are other means of introspection. Complementing these processes the following are useful: identifying past and present prejudices; and identifying past and present approaches to personal problem solving.

2.   Experience:

Personal experiences can also be useful in developing self awarenessin that various facets of our lives offer us opportunities for further learning. This is also known as *experiential learning*, which simply means that we lern from our experiences, i.e through going a particular experience ourselves or by observing others. In this sense experiential learning is a concious process in which we reflect on our personal experience, say in relation to spirituality or lack of it. After this experience (experiential learning), we may achieve a transformation in our knowledge/attitude related to spirituality (see Bernard, 1985) for further guidance on experiential learning and self awareness).

3.   Self awareness through feedback:

Self awareness cannot be developed by adhering solely to the introspection and experiential methods. Introspection and experiential exercises will give us some understanding of ourselves, but a complete self awareness requires knowledge about behaviour too. For this we require the help of others: it takes two to know one fully.

I am aware of my inner feelings (inner processes) but sometimes I cannot see my behaviour. Another person can see my behaviour, but is not aware of my inner feelings and experience. I can see the other person's behaviour, but not his inner experience.

For a complete self awareness, then, we need to reinforce the knowledge gained by introspection, with knowledge obtained by feedback from others about our behaviour.

Self disclosure is a fundamental part of self awareness and it has three characteristics. The disclosures are:

1)   Subjectively true;

2)   Personal statements about self; and

3)   Intentionally revealed to another person.

Self disclosure involves the process of revealing things about yourself (your own ideas, values and feelings) which are similar to those experienced by the person you are trying to help.

There is significant clinical evidence to suggest that a carer's self-disclosure increases the likelihood of the client's self-disclosure (Stuart and Sundeen, 1983). If you talk to them they will talk to you, and often this helps in the therapeutic process. However, our self disclosure must be handled judiciously, and this is determined by the quality, quantity, and appropriateness of what we reveal. We must handle our disclosure sensitively, so that clients feel comfortable enough to tell us something about themselves. If we reveal very little about ourselves, this may reduce the patient's willingness to talk about themselves and, conversely, too many disclosures may decrease the time available for the patient to talk or even alienate him.

COMMUNICATION SKILLS

Good communication skills are a must for spiritual care. The most essential communication skill in spiritual care is active listening without being judgemental. The points about self awareness mentioned earlier are necessary for developing non-judgemental attitudes.

Non-judgemental means unconditional acceptance of others.

However, to have faith, trust and respect for another person despite his behaviour is often a very difficult quality to achieve, but with increasing self awareness it can be developed. A non-judgemental approach is the acceptance of an individual without any kind of judgement, without criticism, and without reservation. This also requires not only unconditional acceptance of a person, but also respect for him/her without necessarily knowing what his/her previous behaviour has been, or who he/she is, because he/she is another human being.

As pointed out earlier, when providing spiritual care, we must reserve or detach from our own personal values, ideals or beliefs. Patients must feel that we are genuinely interested, that we want to know them and how they think and feel, and that we do not judge them. If patients believe that someone else is interested, thinks they are of worth as a unique individuals, and cares about them, then they are far more likely to have a positive image of themselves.

Genuineness is a quality based on the person's ability to be himself or herself. It means being honest and open in expression of our feelings, and not just persons who act the role of nurses. Again, self awareness is a means by which this quality can be developed. It demands honesty and courage to be allowed to be seen as a real person.

Active listening is important because its purpose is to enable the patient to be at ease and to make use of the listening process in such a way that the listener can help the patient deal with spiritual needs and experience further spiritual growth. The active listener acts as a talking mirror, encouraging and reflecting back to the patient what the listener hears, sees, or senses.

The rudiments of being a good listener are as follows:

The carer needs to create the right kind of climate in which the person requiring spiritual care feels accepted and confident enough to be able to talk about his spiritual thoughts and feelings. The patient needs to feel the carer is listening to what he is saying and what he is feeling and not only listening, but accepting and understanding him. All this ties up with responding to people in ways which are helpful. Good listening is really paying close attention to what someone is saying: this is essential, but it is not easy. We need to suspend our thoughts and give the other person our complete attention.

We can demonstrate understanding by reflecting the patient's thoughts back, showing that we are listening hard, that we are making a real effort to understand what the patient is thinking and feeling.

Make the patient feel it is alright to go on talking, that their feelings are being accepted. State that you are genuinely interested in what the patient is saying, and respond warmly.

RUST BUILDING

Trust is necessary because confidence in the nurse-patient relationship is vital in spiritual care and, indeed, to the well-being of the patient. Trust between carer and patient develops over time as the patient tests the environment, risks self-disclosure, and observes the nurse's adherence to commitment.

The following approach enhances initial trust:

- Listening attentively to the patient's feeling.
- Responding to the patient's feelings.
- Demonstrating consistency, especially keeping appointments and promises.
- Viewing the situation from the patient's perspective.

An increasing level of self awareness of personal feelings, along the lines suggested earlier, on the part of the nurse also enhances trust. It enables the patient to disclose uncomfortable, even forbidden, feelings in safety. The nurse must continue to build on the trust gained earlier and this can be achieved by being reliable. Reliability is one other factor that strengthens and sustains a trusting relationship. Reliability is measured in terms of the nurse's commitment to the spiritual needs of the patient and this means promises and adherence to nursing care plans must be carried out promptly and followed through.

GIVING HOPE

Hope is something that we cannot easily give to another, but every effort can be made to support and encourage the hoping abilities of a patient. Nurses often are in ideal positions to foster or hinder hope. A caring relationship can be offered that permit, rather than stifle, the efforts of the patient to develop hope. The nurse can support the person who is testing his own beliefs or struggling with questions of fear and faith. Further encouragement can be given to the patients to talk about their fears. Helping patients to relive their memories is another way of facilitating hoping. Memories of events when life's needs were met, when despair was overcome and when failure was defeated, can all be used to encourage a patient to take a fresh view and face the future with confidence as part of spiritual recovery.

Herth (1990) identifies hope-fostering strategies which could be used as part of spiritual care. She defines hope-fostering strategies as "those sources that functioned to instil, support or restore hope by facilitating the hoping process in some way" (pp. 1253). The following can be utilised as hope-fostering strategies:

Interpersonal connectedness

A meaningful and shared relationship with close ones and others (including carers) is said to be a feature of interpersonal connectedness. For example a harmonious and supportive relationship within the family offers the client hopes and strength which are a fundamental part of a person's spirituality. The willingness of a nurse to share in a patient's hopes is a feature of this strategy.

Light heartedness

The features of this are feelings of delight, joy or playfulness that are communicated verbally or non-verbally. The nurse can foster lightheartedness among patients. The spirit of lightheartedness can provide a communication link between persons and a way of coping with deteriorations in body function and confused emotions; it can provide a sense of release from the present moment.

Personal Attributes

The nurse can enable patients to maximise their attributes of determination, courage and serenity. A search for a sense of inner peace, harmony and calm is one way of enabling the patient to achieve serenity.

Attainable aims

A characteristic of these is the direction of efforts towards some purpose. The presence of aims often foster hope. The nurse who helps patient to search for meaning and purpose in life would actually foster hope. Helping a patient to redefine his aims and channelling his thoughts on to other events or significant others are useful strategies of hope-fostering.

Spiritual Base

The presence of active spiritual beliefs (in God or a 'higher being') and spiritual practices is a source of hope. These can enable patients to participate in specific practices. These may include: praying; enlisting the prayers of others; listening to spiritual music and spiritual programmes on the radio or television; joining in religious activities; maintaining specific religious customs; and receiving visits from members and leaders of their spiritual community.

Uplifting Memories

Recalling uplifting memories and times is another hope-fostering strategy. The nurse can help patients to share happy stories from the past and to reminisce through old picture albums.

Reliving positive activities from the past, such as an enjoyable holiday, significant events (birth of child, receipt of medal) and 'sunset over mountains', can serve to renew the hoping process. It is most likely that memories of past events can serve to enrich the present moment.

Affirmation of Worth

Having one's individuality accepted, honoured and acknowledged can foster hope. Carers, family and friends can be party to a patient's feeling of self worth as a dignified human being. This can be very uplifting and act as a source of hope.

PATIENT EDUCATION

The patient needs to grow spiritually to achieve a full status of health. A good health orientation includes body, mind, spirit and additional consideration of cultural background.

This can be achieved when a nurse creates a relationship in which nurse-patient education takes place. The patient needs to be educated to develop the hoping strategy. Trusting is another skill that can be learned, and the nurse can provide opportunities for the patient to develop this aspect of the relationship. The patient needs learning opportunities to gain insights into his own spiritual awareness. He needs an orientation that would help him to search for meaning and purpose. The nurse as a teacher can help the patient to explore this search for meaning and purpose.

The other aspect of patient education may include the identification of the nature of 'right' relationship with others. Morrison (1990) asserts that nursing concentration on this particular area can lead to improvements in patients' physical health. Educating patients to face up to defective relationships with others is an important aspect of spiritual care. Examples of defective relationships include: the denial of the death of a loved one, a lack of social concern, and an inability to accept hostility. The inability to experience the 'right relationship' is a known cause of spiritual distress (Morrison, 1989).

Learning is seen as a two-way process, in which the patient experiences spiritual growth and the nurse achieves a greater spiritual awareness as well. Millison (1988) found in his study that carers experienced heightened spirituality as a result of their work with ill people, and that all carers reported that they felt they received more in terms of spirituality than they were able to give. An increasing level of knowledge, insight and coping strategies relating to spirituality can be achieved through the two-way process of learning, as mentioned earlier in this section.

SUMMARY

Skills development such as self awareness, communication (listening), trust building, giving hope and patient education is emphasized in this chapter. These skills together with the previous introduction to the knowledge of spirituality offer the reader a basis for the formulation of care plans which include spiritual care. The next two chapters introduce the reader to spiritual care as part of the nursing process.

REFERENCES

BURNARD, P. *Learning Human Skills*, Heinemann Nursing, 1985

HERTH, K. Fostering hope in terminally ill people, *Journal of Advanced Nursing*, 1990, **15**, pp. 1250-1257

MILLISON, M.B., Spirituality and Caregiver, Developing an undertilised facet of care, *The American Journal of Hospice Care*, March/April 1988, pp. 37-44.

MORRISON, R., Spiritual health care and the nurse, *Nursing Standard*, 20 Dec 1989, 4(13/14), pp. 28-29

MORRISON, R., Spiritual health care and the nurse, *Nursing Standard*, 24 Oct 1990, 5(5), pp. 34-35

STUART, G.W. & SUNDEEN, S.J., *Principles and Practice of Psychiatric Nursing*, The C.V. Mosby Company, 1983

Chapter Five:
The Nursing Process and Spirituality

The systematic approach of the nursing process can be employed to assist in meeting the spiritual needs of patients. The following four stages are included in the nursing process: assessment, planning, implementation and evaluation.

ASSESSMENT

Information obtained on religious needs alone is not enough for spiritual care. Such information does not allow us to go deeper into feelings about meaning and purpose of life, love and relationship, trust, hope and strength, forgiveness, expressions of beliefs and values. Also, this approach may lead to the assumption that a person who does not belong to a formal religion has no spiritual needs. As indicated earlier, the non-religious may have spiritual needs. The person who does not express obvious religious beliefs may still struggle with guilt, with lack of meaning and purpose, or with the need for love and relationships. On the other hand, a person who declares allegiance to a particular religion may not necessarily abide by the beliefs and practices of that religion. Assumptions or conclusions should not be drawn about spiritual needs on the basis of patients' religious status.

The nurse must remain sensitive to verbal and non-verbal clues from patients when carrying out spiritual assessment. These clues might indicate a need to talk about spiritual problems.

Assessment of the patient's physical functioning may also provide valuable information for understanding their spiritual component. Such obvious considerations about patient as his ability to see, hear, and move are important factors that may later determine the relevance of certain interventions. Also, psycho-social assessment data may serve a useful purpose in determining the patient's thought patterns, content of speech, affect (mood), cultural orientation, and social relationships, may provide the basis for identifying a need, or planning appropriate care, in conjunction with spiritual intervention.

Stoll (1979) offers a useful guide for spiritual assessment. The guide includes four general areas that can be appraised to derive data about spiritual concerns:

Concept of God or Deity
- Is religion or God significant to you?
- Is prayer (or meditation) helpful to you?

- What happens when you pray (or meditate)?
- Does God or a Deity function in your personal life?
- If yes, can you describe how?
- How would you describe your God or what you worship?

Source of Strength and Hope

- Who is the most important person to you?
- To whom would you turn when you need help?
- Are they available?
- In what ways do they help?
- What is your source of strength and hope?
- What helps you the most when you feel afraid or need special help?

Spiritual Practices

- Do you feel your faith (or religion) is helpful to you?
- If yes, would you tell me how?
- Are there any religious practices that are important to you?
- Has being ill made any difference to your practice of praying (or meditating) or to your other religious practices?
- What religious books or symbols are important to you?

Relation Between Spiritual Beliefs and Health

- What has bothered you most about being sick (or in what is happening to you)?
- What do you think is going to happen to you?
- Has being sick (or what has happened to you) made any difference in your feelings about God or the practice of your faith?
- Is there anything that is especially frightening or meaningful to you now?

Tubesing (1980) suggests a spiritual assessment procedure in which there are five questions to assess a person's spiritual outlook. Spiritual outlook embraces a person's good, faith, value, commitments, and ability to let go and to receive forgiveness from self and others. Tubesing's assessment questions for spiritual outlook are:

- What is the aim of life?
- What beliefs guide me?

- What is important to me?
- What do I choose to spend myself on?
- What am I willing to let go?

The presence of religious literature, for example, the Bible or Koran gives an indication of patient's concerns about spiritual matters. Objects like religious requisites, pins, or articles of clothing are symbolic of patients' spiritual expressions. A patient may keep a religious statue or Deity to carry out his religious rituals. Schedules can be used to carry out spiritual assessment by observation. These are as follows:

Non-verbal behaviour

1. Observe affect. Does the patient's affect or attitude convey loneliness, depression, anger, agitation, or anxiety?

2. Observe behaviour. Does the patient pray during the day? Does the patient rely on religious reading material or other literature for solace?

Verbal behaviour

1. Does the patient seem to complain out of proportion to his illness?

2. Does the patient complain of sleeping difficulties?

3. Does the patient ask for unusually high doses of sedation or pain medication?

4. Does the patient refer to God in any way?

5. Does the patient talk about prayer, faith, hope, or anything of a religious nature?

6. Does the patient talk about church functions that are his life?

7. Does the patient express concern over the meaning and direction of life? Does the patient express concern over the impact of the illness on the meaning of life?

Interpersonal relationships

1. Does patient have visitors or does he/she spend visiting hours alone?

2. Are the visitors supportive or do they seem to leave the patient feeling upset?

3.   Does the patient have visitors from his church?

4.   Does the patient interact with staff and other patients?

Environment

1.   Does the patient have a Bible or other religious reading material with him?

2.   Does the patient wear religious medals or pins?

3.   Does the paient use religious articles such as statues in observing religious practices?

4.   Has the patient received religious get-well cards?

5.   Does the patient use personal pictures, artwork, or music to keep his spirits up?

Observations of the ways in which the patient relates with people "significant others" (people close to him, friends, and others who matter to him) may provide clues to the spiritual needs. The quality of interpersonal relationships can be ascertained. Does the patient welcome his visitors? Does their presence relax the patient or cause distress? Does he get visitors from the church or religious community? Observations of these factors can lead to conclusions about his social support system. The social system enables the patient to give and receive love and lack of such support may deprive the patient of this and leave him distressed. The patient who has faith in God may feel estranged if he is cut off from his support network.

Observations of patient's environment and significant objects/symbols related to his religious practice may give evidence of his spirituality.

The other area of spiritual assessment includes attention to the three factors: sense of meaning and purpose, means of forgiveness, and source of love and relationship. Observations and routine conversations with patients can lead to valuable information about each of those factors. Questions can be framed to include the following:

· What is your source of meaning and purpose in life?
· Why do you go on living?

Observations may include: how does the patient deal with other patients? Does he ruminate over past behaviours or how he has been treated by other people? How does the patient respond to criticisms? If the patient responds with anger, hostility and blames others, these behaviours may suggest that he is unable to forgive himself, and therefore cannot tolerate anything that resembles criticism.

43

The spiritual assessment must also look at the patient's ability to feel loved, valued, and respected by other people.

PLANNING

The planning of spiritual care requires careful attention. The data obtained from assessment must be interpreted in terms of spiritual needs and a care plan should be based on this information. The planning of spiritual care should include: respect for the patient's individuality; willingness of the nurse to get involved in the spirituality of the patient; use of therapeutic self; and the nurturing of the inner person, the spirit.

Assistance to meet spiritual needs should be given according to the indications of the individual, which may be unique and specific. If for example, the patient is part of a church or religious group, and their effect on him appears positive, the nurse can strengthen this contact. A patient who is accustomed to practices such as meditating, praying, or reading the Bible or other religious books, should be given time and privacy. A visit by the patient's religious agent (priest, pastor, rabbi, or others) can be arranged.

The nurse can make it easier for the patient to talk about spiritual beliefs and concerns, especially about how these relate to his illness. The nurse may need to help the patient in his struggle and search for meaning and purpose in life. On the other hand, if the patient is trying to find a source of hope and strength, then it can be used in planning care.

The other aspects of nursing care plan may include comfort, support, warmth, self-awareness, empathy, non-judgemental listening and understanding. All these measures are the essence of a therapeutic relationship. An empathetic listener can do much to support a person who is spiritually distressed by being available when needed, especially those patients suffering from loneliness, and expressing doubts, fears and feelings of alienation. The presence of another empathetic person may have a healing effect. A powerful source of spiritual care and comfort can be prayer, scripture and other religious reading. All these may alleviate spiritual distress. Prayers as a source of help would help a patient develop a feeling of oneness with the universe or a better relationship with God, comfort the patient, and help relieve spiritual distress. A particular prayer should be selected according to each patient's own style of comfort and needs. Although a nurse may not belong to the same faith as the patient, she could still support the patient in carrying out his spiritual acts.

Meditation, both religious and secular can play an important role in enabling patients to relax, clear the mind, achieve a feeling of oneness with a Deity or the universe, promote acceptance of painful memories or decisions, and gather energy and hope that may help them to face spiritual distress. The use of music gives an inspirational and calming effect. A wide variety of religious, inspirational and secular music may spiritually uplift a patient.

IMPLEMENTATION

Implementation of spiritual care is a highly skilful activity. It requires education and experience. Sufficient information is provided in this guide to extend the carer's knowledge of spirituality. In carrying out nursing actions related to spiritual needs, it is imperative that carers observe the following:

- do not impose personal beliefs on patients or families;
- respond to patient's expression of need of a correct understanding of their background;
- do not allow a detached scene to be used as an occasion to proselytise;
- be sensitive to patient's signal for spiritual support.

It is important that if a carer feels unable to respond to a particular situation of spiritual need, then he or she should enlist the services of an appropriate individual.

Nursing intervention should be based on an action which reflects caring for the individual. Caring signifies to the person that he or she is significant, and is worth someone taking the trouble to be concerned about. Caring requires actions of support and assistance in growing. It means non-judgemental approach and showing sensitivity to person's cultural values, physical preference and social needs. It demands an attitude of helping, sharing, nurturing and loving. These actions fulfil the requirement of individualised spiritual care.

An understanding of the patient's unique beliefs and values or religious views is paramount in spiritual care. The carer must respect and understand the need for the patient's beliefs and practices, even if these are not in accord with the nurse's own faith. To allow a better understanding of the patient's spiritual needs, the carer must establish a rapport and trust which makes it easy for the patient to share those beliefs. The carer's own self awareness of personal limitation in understanding these beliefs is paramount and he/she must seek outside help if necessary.

Nursing intervention should be based on a nurse-patient relationship which encourages the person to express views, fears, anxieties, and new understanding through creative acts, writing, poetry, music or art. Time for quiet reflection and opportunities for religious practices would enable the patient to develop a deeper understanding of life and a particular belief system.

The person who has no strong philosophical or religious belief may seek the opportunity to explore feelings, values and an understanding of life with another individual who is willing to give attention and time to discuss those areas of concern and share common human experiences. The nurse is often the person who is most immediately available and receptive to the patient's thoughts and feelings. Certain patients may require their close friends, family or a religious person to share those thoughts and feelings. The nurse must remain sensitive to these needs and make the necessary arrangements. However, it must be remembered that spiritual growth is a life-long process and the nurse who initiates spiritual care will have been a catalyst in the patient's goal to achieve eventual spiritual integrity and well-being.

EVALUATION

Evaluation is an activity that involves the process of making a judgement about outcomes of nursing intervention. There are many indicators of spiritual outcomes, and one of which is spiritual integrity. The person who has attained spiritual integrity, demonstrates this experience through a reality-based tranquillity or peace, or through the development of meaningful, purposeful behaviour. O'Brien (1982) comments that the measure of spiritual care should establish the degree to which 'spiritual pain' was relieved. Another view offered by Kim *et al.* (1984) suggests spiritual care may be measured as the extent to which the 'life principle' was restored. The contents of patient's thoughts and feelings may also reflect spiritual growth through a greater understanding of life, or an acceptance and creativity within a particular context.

As part of evaluation, the following questions may be helpful:

- Is the patient's belief system stronger?
- Do the patient's professed beliefs support and direct actions and words?
- Does the patient gain peace and strength from spiritual resources (such as prayer and minister's visits) to face the rigours of treatment, rehabilitation, or peaceful death?
- Does the patient seem more in control and have a clearer self-concept?
- Is the patient at ease in being alone? in having life plans changed?
- Is the patient's behaviour appropriate to the occasion?
- Has reconciliation of any differences taken place between the patient and others?
- Are mutual respect and love obvious in the patient's relationships with others?

SUMMARY

Effective spiritual care can be given through the systematic steps of the nursing process. Key assessment strategies and tools are indicated in this chapter. Data obtained from assessment strategies can used for planning spiritual care. Practical guidance is provided for implementing spiritual care. Finally, evaluative measures are outlined in determining the patient's spiritual integrity.

REFERENCES

HERTH, K., Fostering Hope in Terminally Ill People, *Journal of Advanced Nursing*, 1990, **15**, pp. 1250-1257

KIM, M.J, McFARLAND, S.K. & McLANE, A.M., *Pocket Guide to Nursing Diagnosis*, C.V Mosby Company, 1984

O'BRIEN, M.E., Religious Faith and Adjustment to Long-term Haemodialysis, *Journal of Religious Health*, 1982, (21), pp. 68.

STOLL, R.G., Guidelines for Spiritual Assessment, *American Journal of Nursing*, 1979, (79), pp. 1574-1577.

TUBESING, D.A., Stress: Spiritual Outlook and Health, *Specialised Pastoral Care Journal*, 1980, (3), pp. 17

Chapter Six:
Putting the Nursing Process into Action

In this chapter examples of specific care plans related to spiritual care are given. Although the focus of care plans outlined in this chapter is on spiritual care it must be remembered that this forms only a part of a more comprehensive holistic care. In order to retain the spiritual focus of this book other aspects of care, though equally important, have been omitted.

Nursing Care in Acute Illness

The spiritual needs of an individual during acute illness are intensified. In acute illness the spiritual needs may reflect as a search for meaning in suffering and death; the patient may feel vulnerable in an impersonal and strange environment, and feel deprived of religious practices which may be a significant way of expressing an individual faith.

The threat of imminent death may accentuate the need for greater spirituality. The fear of death is a universal response no matter how much an individual has prepared for it. The search for meaning becomes more apparent when death has been witnessed by an acutely ill patient who is also anticipating his own death. The non-believer may become bewildered by the absence of any clear meaning and purpose in life. The individual may experience anxiety, doubt, bitterness and fear of the unknown. The person who feels estranged from his family and normal environment and who is suffering pain and fearing death whilst in hospital, may experience the intense need for love and sources of strength and hope. These sources of strength and hope may include family and friends, carers, religious representatives. The person who has a strong religious faith, although relying on sources of strength indicated earlier, also depends ultimately on the love of his God, which may be seen as the greatest gift of all. For some the belief that God is in ultimate control and can provide relief from suffering can be a great source of strength and comfort in enduring pain.

Case History One

Mr John Smith, aged 50, is married with 2 children and works as a self-employed builder. He is generally fit and healthy, a moderate smoker, but with no real vices. John has been taken with severe chest pains to Accident & Emergency by one of his workers . He has now been admitted to the Coronary Care Unit with suspected myocardial infarction. Mr Smith appeared very bewildered by this experience and has become very anxious and frightened. He has no strong religious convictions but belongs to the Church of England.

NURSING CARE PLAN

Problem	Care Plan
Search for meaning and purpose	Listen to patient's feelings and help him to explore meaning and purpose.
Anxiety due to fear of death.	Explore with patient his thoughts and build his hope and expectations.
Estrangement from family and environment.	Help patient: to review his life goals; to recognise family as a source of strength.

Case History Two

Mr Patel, a Hindu, aged 60 years is admitted to a coronary care ward with a history of myocardial infarction. He has now been transferred to a medical ward. He is found to be very distressed and upset whenever he has been visited by his sons.

A nurse found that he had requested his sons to bring a statue of Shiva, his personal Deity, but they had refused because of the fear that the ward staff would object to their father praying to it. It was also found that Mr Patel likes to listen to religious songs and music.

NURSING CARE PLAN

Problem	Care Plan
Distress due to separation from his God and lack of opportunity to carry out his spiritual practices	Build trust. Talk about his feelings. Offer opportunity to carry out religious practices.
Fear of unacceptance and rejection.	Non-judgemental acceptance of beliefs and practices.
Need for relaxation and spiritual inspiration.	Encourage patient to listen to religious songs and music.

Case History Three

Mr Joseph Brown is a 45-year old businessman. He is married, but has no children. He works hard, leading a fairly stressful "executive"-type life, spending time away from home frequently. On one of his business trips, Mr Brown collapses and is admitted to the coronary care unit of the local hospital with a suspected myocardial infarction. His nursing records indicate that he belongs to the Jewish faith. Mr Brown is full of regrets about leading a stressful and busy life and he blames himself for his illness. He also feels distressed that his chances of promotion are going to be affected because of illness and that he will be letting his family down. Mr Brown is worried about his future.

NURSING CARE PLAN

Problem	Care Plan
Love and relationship	Enable patient to believe that his family's love for him is unconditional and not for what or who he is.

Problem	Care Plan
Lack of time for self reflection.	Provide time and space for privacy and self reflection.
Finding a new source of meaning and purpose in life.	Help patient explore meaning and purpose in life.
Expressing faith and religious practices.	Help re-affirm his faith and provide opportunity for expression of faith and to carry out religious practice.
Need for forgiveness; feelings of guilt and self blame.	Encourage patient to talk about his feelings. Strengthen the closeness of family and enable them to act as his source of strength and hope. Build his hope by helping him to review his plans and set new realistic goals for his future plans.

Nursing Care in Chronic Illness

Chronic illness may leave a person in a state of imbalance or disharmony of mind, body and spirit. Feelings of anger, sadness, guilt and anxiety are often common following a period of disorganization and disruption. Despair and hopelessness may loom for the patient and his family. In their struggle with the impact of illness the patient and his family may feel separated from their usual support system. The patient's search for meaning in the disease may become apparent. The patient's adaptation to his illness may mean new resolution, losses to acknowledge, and roles and expectations to be redefined. The illness not only has an impact upon the patient, but his family has to share its effects with him. Although an individuals' reactions to illness differ, many people struggle as a result of the disharmony of mind, body and spirit. For some this means further spiritual growth, for others decline. The impact of an illness on a person compels him to turn in upon himself and re-consider his life (Tournier, 1974).

The illness becomes a spiritual encounter as well as a physical and emotional experience. Research into coping strategies shows that in chronic illness many subjects indicated that they gained strength from their spiritual life (Miller, 1983). The source of strength included a renewed faith in God, prayer, a sense of peace resulting from prayer, and feeling God's love. Other strategies highlighted were meditation, receiving love and support from others, participating in church activities, and a life review.

Case History Four

Mr Robert Smith is aged 65, married and has a diagnosis of carcinoma of the lung. He is a foreman in a local factory. He is being treated with radiotherapy in an oncology ward. He is found to be frequently stating: "Why me? Why has God let this happen to me?" He is angry and bitter towards life generally. He has a strong Christian faith.

NURSING CARE PLAN

Problem	Care Plan
Seeking purpose and meaning of life.	Treat patient with respect and dignity. Enable patient to review his plans and set new future plan.
Needs love and forgiveness.	Encourage patient to talk and help him ventilate his feelings, anger, bitterness and identify source of guilt. Listen with empathy, without being judgemental. Ask chaplain to visit..

Case History Five

Mr Ali Khan, a 52-year old Muslim has a long history of renal disease. He has a small family business. Mr Khan has been admitted to a medical ward following a history of uraemia, unconsciousness and dehydration. He is making a satisfactory recovery but remains very distressed, anxious and expresses feelings of loneliness. His family visit him regularly.

NURSING CARE PLAN

Problem	Care Plan
Spiritual distress due to lack of opportunity for prayer and religious practices.	Build trust and relationship. Listen and encourage patient talk about his needs and faith. Provide privacy and space for prayer and to read the Koran.
Need for love and relationship due to separation from family.	Encourage family to spend time with patient.
Anxiety about not making plans for his family and business.	Help patient to review his plans with his family. Help patient to recognise his family as source of strength.

Nursing Care in Terminal Illness

There is evidence to support spirituality as a significant human experience during terminal illness (Reed, 1987). In some instances a sense of spirituality acts as a resource in terminal illness. Spiritual well-being is related to low death fear, low discomfort, decreased loneliness, emotional adjustment, and positive death perspectives among terminal cancer and other seriously ill patients (Gibbs and Achterberg–Lawlis, 1978; Miller, 1985; O'Brien, 1982). The terminally ill patient facing death is likely to have the following spiritual needs: forgiveness and reconciliation, prayer and/or religious services, spiritual assistance at death, and peace.

Forgiveness and reconciliation

There may be the feeling of unaccomplished relationship in that the patient may not have been granted forgiveness. The patient may seek ways and means of achieving reconciliation and this may reflect as wanting forgiveness and reconciliation with his God. The patient may also need to forgive and be reconciled with others.

Prayer and Religious Services

Prayer, as indicated earlier, can be a source of comfort and strength. Religious services such as receiving sacraments, or blessing of departures, can all be very comforting to the patient and his family.

Spiritual Assistance at Death

The presence of a significant person, such as a doctor, nurse or chaplain at the bedside of a dying patient can be a very comforting spiritual assistance to the patient. This is an invaluable gift that can be given to a dying patient and his family.

Peace

Peace and tranquillity can be achieved through spirituality.

All of the above needs contribute to spiritual well-being and by this means, attainment of peace and tranquillity.

Case History Six

Mr Ronald Clarke, a 50-year old teacher, is married with two teenage children. He has been admitted to hospital in the terminal stages of chronic myeloid leukaemia. He expresses a lot of anxiety about his illness, his wife and children. At times he was found to be frustrated and helpless and full of worries about the future of his family. Although Mr Clarke belongs to the Church of England he has no strong religious beliefs. He likes classical music.

NURSING CARE PLAN

Problem	Care Plan
Anxiety due to separation from his family.	Encourage patient to talk about his feelings.
Frustration because of unachieved tasks in life and incomplete plans concerning security for his family.	Provide time and space for quiet reflection. Give hope by helping patient to revise his plans for the future with his family and set new goals.
Helplessness because of illness	Build patient's hope by uplifting his memories by helping patient to focus on previous achievements, happy events, etc. Help patient to find his family as a source of strength.
Needs opportunity for relaxation.	Provide opportunities for listening to classical music.

Case History Seven

Mrs Murphy, a 75-year old widow was admitted to hospital with terminal carcinoma. She has a strong faith and according to her family she attended a Roman Catholic church frequently and she has been a source of strength to a lot of fellow church goers. In the course of her illness she began to feel agitated, alone and depressed.

NURSING CARE PLAN

Problem	Care Plan
Spiritual distress due to lack of meaning and purpose in life.	Encourage patient to talk about feelings and encourage her to explore meaning and purpose.
Loss of Love and relatedness due to loss of contact with church and friends.	Contact Hospital Chaplain to re-establish contact with church and friends.
Anxiety about not being able to go to church.	Offer opportunity for prayer. Accompany patient to chapel if physical state allows. Contact parish priest

SUMMARY

In each of the above case studies the assessment strategies and tools suggested in Chapter Five can be applied. The care plans outlined in this chapter should not be treated as a precise protocol for spiritual care. Each individual is a unique person and should receive spiritual care as part of individualised patient care, and this cannot be given from a pre-determined formula. The care plans arising from the short case histories are given as an illustration of the points raised earlier in this book. The case histories are chosen to demonstrate the diverse needs of patients from a variety of spiritual and religious background.

REFERENCES

GIBBS, H.W & ARCTERBERG-LAWLIS, J., Spiritual Values and Death Anxiety: Implication for Counselling with Terminal Cancer Patients, *Journal of Counselling Psychology*, 1978, (25), pp. 263-269.

MILLER, J.F., *Coping with Chronic Illness: Overcoming Powerlessness*, F.A Davis, 1983

MILLER, J.F., Assessment of Loneliness and Spiritual Well-being in Chronically Ill and Healthy Adults, *Journal of Psychosocial Nursing*, 1985, pp. 79-85.

O'BRIEN, M.E. Religious Faith and Adjustment to Long-term Haemodialysis, *Journal of Religious Health*, 1982, (21), 68

REED, P.G., Spirituality and Well-being in Terminally Ill Hospitalized Adults, *Research in Nursing and Health*, 1987, **10**(5), pp. 335–344.

TOURNIER, P., *A Doctor's Case Book in the Light of Bible*, 1974, SCM.

Chapter Seven:
Research and Spiritual Care

No book on spiritual care can conclude without a section on research in this area of nursing and this book is no exception. Moreover, readers wishing to research into spiritual care may find this chapter useful, and for many it may serve as a starting point. Concepts related to spirituality are emerging as a result of growing research in this area. Several assumptions are made on the basis of research into the understanding of spirituality. Some of the research findings and assumptions are outlined in this chapter.

Nurses' awareness of spiritual needs.

In a study into nurses' awareness of patients' spiritual concerns, Highfields and Cason (1983) found that although learning opportunities for nurses include content about clients' physical and psychological needs, information about spiritual needs is often omitted. The study found that only patients' expressions of specific beliefs and practices were identified with the spiritual dimension by nurses. Also respondents thought behaviours and conditions related to spirituality occurred infrequently among patients.

The need for nurses to increase their spiritual awareness is stressed by Clifford and Gruca (1987). They write: "Nurses need to start with self-examination of their own spiritual values and attitudes" (pp. 332). Nurses who witness and share in their clients' distress at first hand are likely to become involved in spiritual care.

Spiritual needs of patients

In a survey into spiritual needs, Stallwood (1969) found that many patients would appreciate help in meeting their spiritual needs from a nurse who was available to listen and then personally intervene or refer to the appropriate spiritual counsellor. A further conclusion of this study was that a nurse should also be sensitive to the patient who believes that spiritual care in not the nurse's role and the patient who desires no help at all.

In a descriptive study into spiritual needs, Martin et al. (1976) found that females expressed more spiritual needs than males. Similarly, when Hay (1987) surveyed the general population into their awareness of spirituality, he found that 41% of the women interviewed talked of such experiences, compared with 31% of the men. Martin et al. also found that the clergy is the preferred body with whom patients' prefer to speak about spiritual needs; concerns and kindness were expected from nurses by patients; and nurses were expected to listen to patients.

urse Education and Spirituality

Chadwick (1973) found in her studies that many nurses were aware of the presence of spiritual needs in at least some of their patients, but expressed that they would like further education in meeting spiritual needs in patients. This is consistent with Simsen's (1986) assertion that there is little practical guidance available for nurses who wish to understand a patient's spiritual needs and resources.

In a similar vein, Piles (1986) found in her survey that the role of practising professional registered nurse in providing spiritual care is based on educational preparation for that role. A significant number of those questioned felt inadequately prepared to perform such a role, and many recommended that spiritual care content be included in every basic nursing programme.

pirituality as a basic human need

Burnard (1987) suggests that spirituality is a basic human need and its absence results in spiritual distress. He states: "Spiritual distress is the result of the inability to invest life with meaning. It can be demotivating, fearful and can cause anguish to the sufferer" (pp. 377). He argues that counselling is one approach that can help patient overcome spiritual distress.

pirituality and Mental Illness

According to Peterson and Nelson (1987) in mental illness spiritual distress is related to two phenomena: the inability to practice rituals and the conflict between religious or spiritual beliefs and prescribed health regimes. Both authors suggest that mentally ill clients often struggle with finding a source of meaning and purpose in their lives. The need for forgiveness is a frequent problem in mentally ill clients. Unmet needs in relation to forgiveness result in guilt and resentment.

pirituality and Chronic Illness

In a similar vein, Soeken and Carson (1987) express that a disharmony of mind, body and spirit is a product of the crisis brought on by chronic illness. A period of disorganisation and disruption takes place at the initial stage of adaptation to chronic illness. These authors state: "Following the initial diagnosis of the disease, feelings of sadness, anger, guilt, and anxiety are not uncommon" (pp. 604).

Spirituality and Children

Sommer (1989) suggests children experience spirituality as much as adults. He writes:

> "Who but children can show us so much about what it meant to be human, revealing that all of us are rather fragile creatures, struggling for life, trying to fulfil our potential, expressing our uniqueness, living in relationship with God"

(pp. 225).

Spirituality and Stress

According to Labun (1988) there are interrelationships among the physical, emotional and spiritual aspects of a person. She states: "... stress in the emotional or spiritual aspects may result in a change in physical functioning" (pp. 315). Altered spiritual integrity is reflected as experiences such as spiritual pain, alienation, anxiety, guilt, anger, loss and despair. Spiritual pain can leave a person very distressed and disturbed. Spiritual pain is an experience defined as an individual's perception of hurt or suffering connected with that part of his person that seeks to transcend the realm of the material. It is an experience of a deep sense of hurt stemming from feelings of loss or separation from one's God or Deity, a sense of personal guilt or sinfulness before God or man, a lasting condition of loneliness of spirit (Labun).

Spirituality and Terminal Illness

A study conducted by Reed (1987) revealed that a higher percentage of terminally ill patients had experienced a change and developed an increased level of spirituality than did non-terminally ill or healthy adults. This is consistent with other research findings in which spiritual manifestations of transcendence are significant to the experience faced by the dying patients (Augustine and Kalish, 1975; Bascom, 1984; Hood and Morris, 1983; Klass and Gordon, 1978-79; Lifton, 1979).

SUMMARY

Spirituality as a concept is becoming established as research makes explicit many of its previously unknown facets. Theories and models of spirituality are emerging as a result of research findings. There is now enough research evidence to suggest that spiritual care has a significant place in nursing. It is beyond any doubt that helping patients to meet their spiritiual needs is a fundamental part of holistic care.

REFERENCES

AUGUSTINE, M.J. & KALISH, R.A., Religion, Transcendence, and Appropriate Death, *Journal of Transpersonal Psychology*, 1975, **7**(1), pp. 1–13

BASCOM, G.S., Physical, Emotional, and Cognitive Care of Dying Patients, *Bulletin of Menninger Clinic*, 1984, **48**, pp. 351–356

BURNARD, P., Spiritual Distress and the Nursing Response: Theoretical Consideration and Counselling Skills, *Journal of Advance*, 1987, **12**, pp. 377–382

CHADWICK,R., Awareness and Preparedness of Nurses to Meet Spiritual Needs *In* SHELLY, A. & FISH, S. (Eds.) *Spiritual Care: The Nurse's Role*, InterVarsity Press, 1983, pp. 177–178.

CLIFFORD, B.S. & GRUCA A., Facilitating Spiritual Care, *Rehabilitation Nursing*, Nov-Dec 1987, **12**(6), pp. 331–333.

HAY, D., *Exploring Inner Space*, Mowbray, 1987

HIGHFIELDS, M.F. & CASON C., Spiritual Needs of Patients: Are they recognised?, *Cancer Nursing*, June 1983, pp. 187–192

HOOD,R.W., Jr., & MORRIS, R.J, Toward a theory of death transcendence, *Journal for the Scientific Study of Religion*, 1983, **22**, pp. 353-365.

KLASS,D & GORDON, A. Varieties of Transcending Experience at Death: a Videotape-based Study, *OMEGA*, 1978-79, **9**, pp. 19–36

LABUN, E., Spiritual Care: an Element in Nursing Care Planning, *Journal of Advanced Nursing*, 1988, **13** pp. 314–320.

LIFTON, R.J., *The Broken Connection*, Simon and Schuster, 1979

MARTIN, C., BURROWS, C. & POMILLOIO Spiritual Needs of Patients Study, *In* SHELLY, A. & FISH, S. (Eds.) *Spiritual Care: The Nurse's Role*, InterVarsity Press, 1988, pp. 160-176.

PETERSON, E. & NELSON, K. How to Meet your Clients' Spiritual Needs, *Journal of Psychosocial Nursing*, May 1987, Vol 25, No 5, p 34-38.

PILES, C. *Spiritual Care: Role of Nursing Education and Practice: a needs survey for curriculum development* unpublished doctoral dissertation. St Louis University, 1986

REED, P.G. Spirituality and Well-being in Terminally Ill Hospitalised Adults, *Research in Nursing and Health*, 1987, **10(5), pp. 335–344**

SIMSEN,B., The Spiritual Dimension, *Nursing Times, Nov 1986, (26), p 41-42*

SOEKEN, K.L & CARSON, V. J., Responding to the Spiritual Needs of the Chronically Ill, *Nursing Clinics of North America*, Sept 1987, **22**(3), pp. 603–611.

SOMMER, D.R. The Spiritual Needs of Dying Children, *Issues in Comprehensive Pediatric Nursing*, 1989, **12**(2–3), pp. 225–233.

STALLWOOD, J., Spiritual Dimensions of Nursing Practice *In* BELAND, I. & PASSOS, J. (Eds.) *Clinical Nursing*, Macmillan, 1975.

Further Reading Guide

Readers wishing to carry out small- or large-scale research into spiritual care will find the following books useful:

BURNARD, P. and MORRISON, P., *Developing Basic Skills*, Macmillan, 1990.

An excellent book written by nurse educators for nurses, which offers a jargon-free, step-by-step guide to doing nursing research. It is full of activity-based learning units and resource materials for researchers (beginners to advanced).

CALNAN, W., *Coping with Research*, William Heinemann Medical Books, London, 1984

A practical and easy-to-read guide to research for beginners.

Index